SEVEN KEYS TO UNLIMITED PERSONAL ACHIEVEMENT

Author: Terry Lemerond

Forward by Mark Victor Hansen

Co-Author of the #1 New York Times best selling series,

Chicken Soup for the Soul

Change your beliefs, change your life

Published by:

Dogwood Press

Over the years, other people have shared with me life-changing ideas on positive thinking, visualization, affirmations, goal-setting, and dealing with setbacks. I have read literally thousands of books and listened to thousands of tapes and CD's in order to absorb this wisdom and use it in my own life. The insights of others have helped me mold my life the way I want it to be. They have helped me "sculpt" my very self so I can be the person I want to be. Granted, I'm not all the way there, but I'm pretty sure I'm on the right path.

I am not a motivational speaker or a professional writer. I own a dietary supplements company in Green Bay, Wisconsin. So what does a vitamin company have to do with belief?

Actually, it has everything to do with belief. Almost 40 years ago, I made myself believe I could run my own business, and—with the help of a generous woman named Claire Delsmann—I bought a health food store. Almost 40 years ago, I started believing I could develop nutritional formulas to support specific functions of the body, and several nutrition companies were born. I then believed my colleagues and I could build this fledgling operation into a thriving, international business. As you read this book, we now have developed products that can be found in health food stores all over the world.

The greatest blessing

Am I luckier than other people? I doubt it. Am I smarter? Not necessarily. Did I inherit a lot of money? Not even close.

Truly, my life has been blessed. But God didn't hand me a growing company, gifted and hard-working employees, and a satisfying personal life. What God did give me was the gift of belief. I found that the more I believed, the closer I got to my goals. It was belief that led me to attempt certain ventures, to read inspiring books, to choose the right friends. It was belief that kept me going in the face of daunting obstacles. It was belief that kept me close to God, because I believed God would never abandon me. I was right.

There is no way I could have accomplished what I have in life without God. I owe everything to God, and I will always be grateful for His abundant blessings.

Sharing whatever I can

In my first book, *Seven Keys to Vibrant Health*, I focused on approaches to physical and mental well-being. These included spirituality, positive attitude, exercise, diet, supplementation, and more.

In this booklet, I want to delve a little deeper. What do you need to make the right choices? What's the prerequisite to living your life to the fullest? Belief. Your beliefs are your reality.

I'm not approaching you as an expert in the field. I haven't formally studied psychology or motivation. I just know what worked for me. And the ideas you'll find in the following pages certainly did not originate with me. I am following in the footsteps of many fine writers and thinkers: Norman Vincent Peale, Jack Hartman, Mark Victor Hansen, Dennis Waitley, Anthony Robbins, Zig Ziglar, Earl Nightingale, and Brian Tracy are just a few.

The level of success we reach reflects the kind of people we surround ourselves with. By teaming up with brilliant, courageous, caring, and magnificent people, we become better ourselves.

My friendship with Captain Vito was the start of an important life change for me. The books, tapes and CD's I've "soaked up" over the years continued to nourish my growth. I have received much that is good in my life. Now I want to give something back. This booklet is my expression of gratitude to the many people who've supported my journey.

Seven Keys to Unlimited Personal Achievement is based on actual experience. I know these precepts are powerfully effective because they are working for me and for many of the people I know. When you apply the "keys" you find here, you will be amazed at the way the universe opens up to you. This is not abstract, pie-in-the-sky theory. This is fact. Try it and watch it all happen for you.

And start believing.

Terry Lemerond

Contents

Dedication

*This book is dedicated to my three wonderful grandchildren,
Roman, Angelique and Anna.*

*And Jesus
I can do all things through Christ who gives me the strength*

*Jesus said unto him, If thou canst believe, all things are
possible to him that believeth.*
Mark 9:23

Foreword

When I first met Terry Lemerond, I felt an immediate connection. What struck me was his enthusiasm, determination, and courage to pursue his dreams. His energy was contagious and his warmth was genuine.

Terry is an impeccable man, a visionary leader, company executive, and a friend. I love, trust, respect, and admire him.

He has transformed himself from sickness to health, from rags to riches, and from a shy and insecure man to a powerful, influential, and charismatic leader.

The future of the world is definitely better off, because Terry has a vision that everyone can choose to become radiantly healthy, happy, and enjoy the experience of self-fulfillment.

I admire Terry's success: He came from a modest background to become president of a thriving natural supplements company, host of a popular national radio talk show, and widely read author. But even more than his worldly success, I have been impressed with what lies within Terry. He lives life with a passion: a passion for God, his family, his vocation, and for anyone who wants to make their life a joyful, glorious experience filled with success and prosperity.

Motivation has fascinated Terry for most of his adult life. He once told me that if he hadn't been so passionate about the natural health field, he would have been a motivational speaker. He credits other motivational speakers and writers for his success and personal happiness. They gave him the necessary tools for reaching his goals.

In this easy-to-read booklet, Terry talks directly to you. He includes stories, his own experience, and the writings of others to show how you can make your life richer, deeper, and more successful on every level. This philosophy worked for him; he knows it'll work for you, too.

Mark Victor Hansen
coauthor of the #1 New York Times best-selling series,
Chicken Soup for the Soul

Introduction

Change your beliefs and you change your life

Have you ever wondered why one person is successful and another isn't? Two people may have the same level of talent, the same IQ, the same education, the same advantages. And yet one is a CEO of a thriving corporation, and the other collects unemployment checks. Is it luck? Is it fate? Does God favor one over the other?

I've watched a lot of people over the years: the successful and the unsuccessful, those who fulfill their dreams and those who only talk about it, those who overcome difficult obstacles and those who bitterly complain about them. I am convinced that the difference between winners and losers is belief. What we believe comes true. Winners believe the world is wide open to them, and losers believe that the world has shut them out. They are both correct.

I had to change my beliefs, too

Belief has made a big difference in my own life. When I was a young man, I was sarcastic and miserable. I believed nothing mattered, so I ate poorly, didn't exercise, and became grossly overweight. I believed I couldn't make friends, and I didn't. I believed I wouldn't like the jobs I was hired for, and—what do you know—I didn't. I believed I was of no use to anyone, and at that time, it was probably true.

What changed? My beliefs. I joined the Marine Corps where I met and befriended Captain Ed Vito. He taught me the importance of good health, proper nutrition, and regular exercise. Oddly enough (from my perspective), he actually believed in me. That helped me believe in myself. I began to work out, lose my excess weight, eat more healthfully, and actually feel good. With a sense of awe, I finally believed I could change my life. With plenty of help and moral support, I transformed myself from a pudgy, churlish, and aimless teenager into a physically fit, self-confident, and focused young man.

Passing the torch

Now that I have met many of my goals, I want to do the same favor for someone else—for you. That's why I wrote this book. And then, when these ideas start working for you, you can pass them on to someone else. Let's continue this positive chain reaction.

1

Becoming the best we can be

In 1969, when I became the owner of Bay Natural Foods in Green Bay, Wisconsin, my goal was to make $85 a day in sales. It was a modest goal, and we quickly reached it.

With each success, my goals became a little bigger, a little bolder. I dreamed of developing my own products. I dreamed of creating my own company. I dreamed of entering a global market. I dreamed of writing a book.

Each of these dreams came true. I don't tell you this in order to boast. What I want to do is illustrate the necessity of setting goals. When we discover what we want our lives to become, when we take concrete, specific steps to get there, we begin to accomplish amazing things. You only have to try it to find out for yourself.

What is life without goals?

We've all known people without goals. Because they never plan their tomorrows, they never fully live their todays.

Perhaps these individuals have plenty of potential, but no direction. And when intelligence and talent and energy gets turned inward, it creates a frustrated, bitter, and unlikable human being. They may belittle the accomplishments of others because they themselves have nothing positive to contribute.

In *Being the Best*, Denis Waitley writes, "...aimless living is like traveling on a ship without a rudder...purposeless, rudderless living leads to the frustration of negative attitudes and poor self-esteem."

Tony Robbins, well-known motivational speaker and author of *Unlimited Power: New Science of Personal Achievement* and *Awaken the Giant Within*, explains it this way: You may be an expert marksman, but that only has meaning if you have a target.

Take time to dream

Before you begin to set goals, you need to allow yourself to dream. What have you always wanted to do? What kind of person do you want to become? How do you see yourself in five years? Ten years? Thirty years? This may sound simple, but too few people truly understand their own desires. As Alfred E. Newman, the *MAD* magazine character said, "Most people don't know what they want, but they're pretty sure they haven't got it!"

Perhaps we think of dreaming as childish or self-indulgent. But I believe that without dreams, we are destined to skim the surface of life rather than plunging into its fascinating and endless depths. Joe Batten, author of *Expectations and Possibilities*, writes, "A dream is that most precious part of us that is personal, unique and real."

Identify your purpose

It's also important to have a unifying purpose for your various life goals. That purpose may be spiritual, humanitarian, educational, or financial. Mark Victor Hansen and Jack Canfield, authors of *Dare to Win*, write that "A purpose is the underlying direction that gives meaning to our goals…leaves attached to a growing tree have the purpose of keeping that tree alive and healthy." In contrast, they compare indiscriminate and undirected goals to fallen leaves that are easily scattered by the wind.

Believe in yourself!

After you've allowed yourself to dream and you've identified your purpose, you must absolutely believe you can achieve your goals. As Tony Robbins says, "Success or failure begins with a belief. Whether you believe you can do something or you believe you can't, you're probably right."

Successful people believe in themselves, even in the face of failure and rejection. The great artist Renoir was told over and over again to give up painting because he had no talent. He continued because he believed in his own gift, and now his masterpieces hang in museums throughout the world. He didn't allow anyone else to convince him of something he knew in his heart was not true.

Robbins explains that once you tell yourself you can't do something, you turn off the neurological pathways that would have made it possible. On the other hand, when you tell yourself you *can* do something, you open up those pathways that provide the resources for accomplishment.

Write it down

Thinking about goals is only the first step. It's essential to write down clear, specific goals. Consider this: A study found that only three percent of 1953 Yale graduates had written down clear, specific goals. Twenty years later, the researchers interviewed the surviving members of the 1953 graduating class. That small percentage who'd written down their goals were worth more financially than the other 97 percent put together. More importantly, this three percent also reported a higher level of happiness.

Getting there

In *Unlimited Power*, Tony Robbins provides 12 clear steps for reaching your goals. I'll summarize them here:

1. Make an inventory of your goals, without any limits. Take a pen and write nonstop for 10 or 15 minutes.
2. Go over your list and estimate when you expect to reach those goals. Next week? In ten years?
3. Pick out the four most important goals for this year. Write down why you will achieve them. Be clear and positive.
4. Evaluate your key goals. Are they positive? Specific? How will you know when you've achieved these goals? Are they within your control? Are the goals ecologically sound and desirable? If you can't answer these questions satisfactorily, perhaps you should reconsider your goals.
5. Make a list of the resources already available to you. They may include character traits, friends, money, education, and energy.
6. Focus on the times you used some of these resources successfully. Describe what you did that made you succeed, and what about the experience made you feel successful.
7. Describe the kind of person you'd have to be to reach your goals. What are the characteristics, skills, attitudes, beliefs, and disciplines you'd need to accomplish them?
8. Write down what prevents you from reaching your goals. Do you fail to plan? Fail to act? Do too many things at once? Become paralyzed with doubt and fear?
9. Create a step-by-step plan for each of your key goals. The plans must include something you can do today.

10. Write down the names of three to five people who've achieved what you want to achieve. What made them successful? What advice might they give you?
11. Create your ideal day. What would you do? Where would you be? What people would be involved? Plan it out, from the time you get up to the time you go to sleep.
12. Describe your perfect environment for success. Outside or inside? What tools would you have? What support people would you have to help you?

These steps will help you clarify exactly what you want and how you can get it.

Manageable steps

Keep in mind that every journey begins with a single step. Big goals are more achievable when they're broken down into small steps. For example, when I wrote *Seven Keys to Vibrant Health*, I didn't just sit down and write 113 pages. I wrote a sentence at a time. The sentences became paragraphs. The paragraphs became whole pages. The pages became chapters. The chapters became an entire book. Bit by bit, I achieved a goal that had once seemed almost more than I could hope for.

Take risks

Setting goals is risky. It requires you to take action and prove your mettle. You may fear that you won't achieve your goals and that you'll feel like a loser. You may fear that it will be difficult to reach for something you want. And that's the whole point!

The only way to discover new strengths, talents, and possibilities is to face problems and deal with obstacles. Life's challenges force us to stretch, to try something new, to be more than we were before. And apparently, that is the very key to happiness. After an extensive, year-long study on happiness, researcher Dr. Henry C. Link concluded, "Virtually every day of his life, the happy American does, or attempts to do, something difficult."

What about security? Joe Batten writes in *Expectations and Possibilities* that when we retreat into ourselves for safety and low-risk living, we begin to atrophy and die.

Besides—as Denis Waitley points out in *Being the Best*—total security is a myth. Life is full of unexpected illnesses, accidents, tax audits, job layoffs, bankruptcy, even terrorists. We cannot protect ourselves from all of life's perils.

On the other hand, if our goal is to live fully—not just securely—we enjoy more opportunities for love, satisfying work, financial success, and self-fulfillment.

For ten years, I worked at a machine shop, and I hated every moment of it. It just wasn't for me. But I had a family to support, so I stuck with it. When I took over Bay Natural Foods, I was taking a big risk because I wasn't sure what the future held.

If I had not taken that risk, I would be an angry and unfulfilled man today. As it turned out, that risky venture changed my life in phenomenal ways. I thank God for giving me the courage to swallow my fears and take the jump. I have never once looked back.

Gratitude

Finally, it's important to focus on not just what we want, but what we already have. We shouldn't become so obsessed with our goals that we don't appreciate our past and present achievements. Tony Robbins recommends keeping a gratitude diary of former goals we have already accomplished.

I feel I have been greatly blessed, and I thank God for these blessings every day of my life. I have a loving family, supportive and nurturing friends, a growing business, and excellent health.

And yet, I'm still setting goals. If dreaming of possibilities has gotten me this far today, who knows how far I can go in the long run? Do you know how far you can go?

Let's find out.

2

When you visualize what you want, you're one giant step closer

Visualization? What's *that?* Well, I'll start by telling you what it's not. Visualization is not idle daydreaming and it's not a waste of time.

Visualization is a powerful tool you can use to focus your mind, harness your energies, combat stress and illness, and get exactly what you want in life.

For example, Brian Boitano used visualization to win the 1988 Olympic Gold Medal for figure skating. He said, "It was my dream performance that I've visualized a million times, at least once a day, since I was nine years old."

When you visualize, you "see" a specific, concrete result. You use your imagination to transform vague dreams into vivid mental realities. Visualization may be unconscious, or it may be a part of guided meditation. Conscious, controlled visualization is absolutely necessary if you're serious about reaching your goals.

How to visualize

The following guidelines come from *Psycho-Cybernetics: A New Technique for Using Your Subconscious Power*, by Maxwell Maltz, M.D.

Dr. Maltz recommends setting aside a half hour each day when you can be alone and uninterrupted. You need to completely relax and make yourself comfortable. Close your eyes and release your imagination. "You want your mental pictures to approximate actual experience as much as possible," he writes. "The way to do this is to pay attention to small details, sights, sounds, objects, in your imagined environment."

During this 30 minutes, Dr. Maltz advises, see yourself acting and reacting in a successful and ideal way. For example, if you are typically shy and nervous, envision yourself as confident and poised among people. Imagine what you are wearing, how you are moving, what you are saying.

Dr. Maltz explains that this exercise builds new "memories" in your brain and central nervous system. After you practice it for awhile, you are likely to find yourself acting exactly the way you have imagined—and seemingly without effort. When these confident, competent images are finally transformed into an automatic mechanism, your vision becomes spontaneous and real.

In his book, Dr. Maltz cites the wisdom of Dr. Harry Emerson Fosdick: "Hold a picture of yourself long and steadily enough in your mind's eye and you will be drawn toward it," states Dr. Fosdick. "Picture yourself vividly as winning and that alone will contribute immeasurably to success."

Making yourself well

The power of visualization extends far beyond professional or financial success or relaxation. It can actually improve your health. *Your Body Believes Every Word You Say,* by Barbara Hoberman Levine, claims, "...visualization can help destroy bacteria and viruses, reduce tumors, heal broken bones and restore organic function in any part of the body."

Can we simply *tell* the body to get well? Not according to Kenneth Pope of the Brentwood, California Veterans Administration hospital. At the first annual conference on mental imagery, he said, "Telling your blood pressure to drop just doesn't do it...the autonomic nervous system responds to a more basic language—imagery."

Pope reported the results of a study in which hypertensive patients using visualization plus relaxation techniques reduced their blood pressure more effectively than those who used relaxation alone. The visualization group actually pictured their blood vessels widening.

Devouring cancer cells

Here's another compelling example of the therapeutic potential of visualization: Erik Esselstyn was suffering from bile duct cancer. Instead of giving up, he began to visualize an army of white polar bears fighting his cancer. "I saw countless imaginary polar bears coursing through my bloodstream and lymphatic system, always on the lookout for cancer cells, always ready to devour them."

Esselstyn reported that for the two years following his surgery, he could sense the "polar bears" eating up the cancer cells. Each time, he felt certain more cancer cells had been conquered. At the conclusion of each visualization session, the triumphant polar bears gathered at the top of his brain with their thumbs up for victory. The malignancy never came back.

Barbara Hoberman Levine also suggests imagining other symbolic warriors to fight off infections, allergies, cancerous growths or tumors. These could be white knights, doctors, warfare weapons, tanks, garbage trucks, or squirt guns. Or, if you prefer a less adversarial approach, Levine recommends weapons of love, such as valentines or a laser beam of golden light.

Citing a study on cancer patients, Dr. Rossman pointed out that even when visualization did not cure the disease, patients reported relief from anxiety and pain, greater tolerance of chemotherapy or radiation, and improved ability to cope with the illness. They claimed that imagery decreased stress and helped them feel more in control of their lives.

After all, there's more to healing than a medical cure. There's a healing of the spirit—the most powerful healing of all.

Visualization for good or bad

The Bible says, "The wicked man's fears will all come true, and so will the good man's hopes."

Unfortunately, much of the unconscious visualization we do is negative. We get into the self-destructive habit of visualizing ourselves bumbling through a job interview, or getting into a car accident, or having a terrible fight with our spouse. That doesn't make us "wicked," but it does put our energies into all the wrong directions.

Shakti Gawain, author of *Creative Visualization*, writes, "We often imagine limitations, difficulties, and problems—and that's what we get."

What you visualize is entirely within your power. For example, you can choose to visualize yourself walking into a prospective employer's office with your head up and your shoulders back. Imagine that your handshake is firm and confident. Hear yourself answering questions articulately. Imagine asking intelligent and appropriate questions. "See" yourself as absolutely, without a doubt, the best candidate for the job.

Will visualization guarantee you a job? Of course not. But it will guarantee that you'll go into your interview with higher expectations of the experience and of yourself. And when you expect success, you're far more likely to find success.

Putting your energies in the right directions

Positive visualization can strengthen all areas of your life. Visualize a loving encounter with your spouse or child or friend. Visualize yourself finishing a marathon. Visualize yourself getting rid of unwanted body fat. As you create these favorable images and sensations in your own mind, you are pouring your energy into these desirable realities.

Gawain explains that the physical universe is actually energy, and that we are all part of a single, vast energy field. She says that thoughts and feelings have a magnetic energy which draws energy of a similar nature. "We can see this principle at work, for instance, when we 'accidentally' run into someone we've just been thinking of, or 'happen' to pick up a book which contains exactly the perfect information we need at that moment," Gawain writes.

In other words, it is no accident. What we create in our minds, we create in our lives.

Conquering the fear of visualization

The concept of visualization makes some people uneasy. They may fear the unknown, or they may be reluctant to face the feelings that emerge. However, our feelings cannot hurt us. The only thing that can keep us from moving ahead is our fear of those feelings.

If a disturbing feeling surfaces during creative visualization, "...the best thing is simply to look at it fully, be with it and experience it as much as you can, and you will find that it loses any negative power over you," Gawain writes.

Of course, you cannot *act* on all feelings, but you can acknowledge that they exist. And when you are no longer a stranger to yourself, you feel a lot more comfortable inside your own skin.

Understanding yourself through visualization

Visualization can be profoundly enlightening. When you engage in creative visualization, you begin to face your most fundamental attitudes. You find out what's holding you back, what stops you from getting what you desire in life. Once you recognize these destructive habits of thought, you can banish them through constructive visualization.

Taking control of your life and your future

Visualization takes practice: The more you do it, the easier it becomes, and the more results you reap. You can use visualization to achieve goals, to reduce stress, and even to heal yourself.

And there's a bonus: Visualization costs you nothing. It has no side effects. You can do it alone or in a crowd. And it is proof that the intangible imagination can create tangible realities.

Everything you want in life starts in your mysterious and powerful mind. The only limitations are the ones you have created. And what you have created, you can change. It's entirely your choice.

3

Affirmations:
Talking yourself into a better reality

Admit it: You talk to yourself. We all do. And the important question isn't whether you talk to yourself or not, it's what you tell yourself. If you're giving yourself the message, "I'm failing," you're automatically increasing your chances for failure. Conversely, when you tell yourself, "I'm succeeding," you're well on your way to success.

Just as negative statements often become self-fulfilling prophecies, so do positive statements. It may sound simplistic, but I truly believe that we can talk ourselves into greater accomplishments, more satisfying relationships, and better health.

Affirmations are a powerful tool that can help you lead a more fulfilling life. However, making them an automatic part of your thought processes is challenging. It takes persistence and determination to replace negative affirmations with positive ones. But if you're serious about taking control of your life and your world, conscious affirmations are a step in the right direction.

What seeds are you planting?

When we plant statements in our minds, we're like a farmer who plants seeds. He or she uses certain tools to prepare the soil. The farmer understands that the crop requires patience, time, watering, and weeding.

We do the same thing with the garden of our mind. We either plant a harmful weed or a seed of greatness. Whatever we plant in our psyche eventually germinates.

Words have enormous power. Words can create or destroy. And the words we say to ourselves often become true.

The destructive power of negative statements

Unfortunately, most people's messages to themselves are put-downs.

And it's no wonder: Children receive a mere 32 positive messages a day and an overwhelming 427 negative ones. If we grow up hearing, "that was stupid," we internalize it so the message becomes, "I am stupid." Too often, this critical self-talk becomes a habit, and we're barely aware of our own semi-conscious, running commentary: "I'm ugly. That person will never go out with me. I'll never graduate. They'll never hire me. I'm not good enough to get that promotion. I can't afford the kind of house I want to live in."

Stuart Wilde, author of *Affirmations*, writes that the mind often seeks limitations and restrictions. Limitations enclose us with boundaries that make us feel safe. Negative self-talk may actually become comfortable in its familiarity.

But this familiarity can be stifling and self-destructive. According to Julia Cameron, author of *The Artist's Way: A Spiritual Path to Higher Creativity,* these core negative beliefs keep us scared. "They attack your sexuality, lovability, intelligence—wherever you're most vulnerable," she writes. "But these negative feelings are not facts—they are only beliefs. We need to confront them and correct them."

How I turned my life around

When I was growing up, I was a very negative and unhappy person. I squandered an awful lot of energy on worry, anxiety, hostility, and depression. I believed terrible things about myself, and simply couldn't accept any positive feedback people would try to give me. I kept expecting the worst to happen—and it often did. It wasn't until I started planting positive messages, started expecting better things to happen, that my life began to turn around.

How did I change? I have read literally thousands of books and I listen to self-improvement tapes almost all the time. I keep saturating my life with positive input and positive people. Just as we need to nourish and exercise the body, we need to nourish and exercise the mind with uplifting and optimistic influences. We have to replace old, destructive messages with new, hopeful messages. The more we repeat these new messages, the faster they become our new reality.

Importance of self-esteem

The quality of your life depends on your self-esteem. If you're paralyzed with self-loathing, how do you face each new day? How do you take the necessary risks to achieve your goals? How can you treat yourself with the affection and respect you truly deserve?

We all face setbacks in life. Failures, in themselves, are not problems; they can be challenges to succeed. But if we react to failure by putting ourselves down, we create a problem.

The person with low self-esteem will react to a setback with, "I'm such a loser. Why should I even try again? I'll only screw it up." In contrast, a person with high self-esteem can shrug off adversity, seeing it as just one step toward success. For example, a nonconformist group of artists was once ostracized from the established art community, who believed these "upstarts" had no talent. However, Degas, Pissarro, Monet, Cézanne, and Renoir continued working, because they believed in their own genius. And now the world does, too.

In *Seeds of Greatness*, author Denis Waitley points out that "You are your most important critic. No opinion is so vitally important to your well-being as the opinion you have of yourself."

To promote a healthy self-esteem, take a detailed inventory of your strengths, assets, and attributes, suggests Zig Ziglar in *See You at the Top*. Did you successfully graduate from high school? College? Are you proficient at your job, whether it be meter reader, computer programmer, or CEO? Are you a good neighbor? A good friend? Did you give up smoking? Have you overcome other difficulties? Do you contribute to charities or volunteer your time and talents? Do people enjoy your sense of humor? When you start to look at your life and yourself, you may be amazed at all the good you'll find.

What to tell yourself

Affirmations are highly personal, and you need to develop ones that specifically work for you. Here are some examples:
"I am unique and special."
"I am feeling greater physical health and vitality."
"I am reaching my financial goals."
"I deserve a rich and rewarding creative life."
Here are a few of my own:
"I can do all things through Christ who strengthens me."
"Love flows through me in avalanches of abundance."

When you're developing your own affirmations, the following tips may help: State them in the present tense, phrase them as positive statements, keep them short and direct, and try to fully experience what you are affirming.

When you give yourself positive affirmations, you're instructing your subconscious to become your ideal self, explains Mark Victor

Hansen and Jack Canfield in *Dare to Win*. When you declare these affirmations, you have to make sure you live up to them. In addition, when you become convinced of your affirmations, you convince others, too.

Affirming others

Naturally, affirmations are not for you alone. Every individual on the face of this planet needs to be acknowledged. We desperately want to be recognized for our integrity, kindness, courage, self-discipline, wit, determination or capacity for loving.

In *Dare to Win*, Hansen and Canfield point out that when we sincerely affirm another human being, we raise that person's self-esteem as well as our own. We can affirm others for their mental attributes, their character, their achievements, or their behavior. Usually, that person will reciprocate, so we come out ahead, too.

"Affirm everyone you meet," the authors recommend. "It will help them immensely in their lives, and it will come back to you in many positive and often unseen ways."

By reaching out to others in a caring way, we're actually caring for ourselves, too.

Affirmations take practice

Like any new skill, positive affirmations may feel strange and awkward at first. Most of us have an inner censor that automatically objects to affirmations, according to writer and artist Julia Cameron. For example, when we tell ourselves we can make a decent living and follow our dreams, our inner censor is likely to respond with, "Who do you think you are? Get your head out of the clouds and find a real job!"

Cameron urges us to find the root of our inner censor. Was it an over-cautious parent? A belittling teacher? A mentor with too little vision? Once we track down the origin of our internal censor, Cameron suggests, we drain its power.

It may feel odd, at first, to tell ourselves that we are worthwhile, that we deserve health, success, love and happiness, that we are talented and capable. We have to stick with it until these positive statements no longer feel uncomfortable. All at once, we realize that what we've been telling ourselves has actually turned into indisputable reality. We have talked ourselves into the kind of life we have always wanted to have, into becoming the kind of person we have always wanted to be.

And when we reach this point, we realize that this is no less than we deserve.

4

Shatter your limits!

From the day we're born, others try to limit us. Some of the limits are sensible: Our parents didn't want us to walk into traffic or burn our hand on a hot stove. But some of the limits were set more out of fear than common sense. Perhaps you heard, "Oh, you're a girl, you'll never excel at math," or, "You're too small, you'll never be a really good athlete."

I don't think our parents meant to sabotage our success; I believe they were trying to save us from failure and disappointment. But in doing so, they may have unintentionally blocked us from our full potential, from seeing for ourselves how much we could do and how far we could go.

When I decided to run my own business almost 30 years ago, my mother warned me against it. She did it with the best intentions: She didn't want to see me get hurt. As it turned out, her fears were unfounded. That single decision opened up a whole new life for me. I love and respect my mother, but I'm glad I didn't internalize the limits she attempted to set.

Danger of internalizing limits

Long after parents and others have stopped imposing limits on us, we may do the job ourselves. Instead of Mom and Dad telling us, "You're not smart enough to go to college," or "Why try losing weight? You know you'll always be fat," we start giving ourselves these messages.

I'd like to tell you a true story about internalizing limits. There was an aspiring writer who tossed his first completed book manuscript into the trash. He told himself that he had no talent and that his writing was junk. However, his wife believed in him more than he did. She fished his manuscript out of the garbage, sent it to several

15

publishers, and finally found someone to publish it. The book was *Carrie*, Stephen King's first.

Since we don't all have spouses who'll push those limits for us, we need to do it for ourselves. If it weren't for these limits—self-imposed or otherwise—imagine what we could do!

When your limits disappear...

When we don't realize something is impossible, we may discover incredible possibilities. For example, there was a college student in a math class who fell asleep. He woke up at the end of class and saw two math problems on the blackboard. He assumed this was his homework, so he copied the problems down and took them home. For the next couple of days, he struggled mightily with these difficult problems. He eventually solved the first one, but couldn't find an answer to the second.

Finally, in frustration, the young man consulted his professor. "I have to apologize," he said. "I fell asleep in your class, and when I tried to do the homework you assigned, I was only able to answer one of the problems." The professor was shocked and pulled the homework out of the student's hands.

After examining the homework, the professor said, "You're right; you answered the first problem. But I had just explained to the class that both of these problems were unsolvable. No one has ever been able to figure them out."

Since our student didn't know the problems were unsolvable, he achieved the impossible.

A movie titled *The Miracle Man* features a real-life hospital patient who broke his neck. He was told he would never be able to eat on his own, use the bathroom on his own, or walk again. He refused to believe it. He said, "I will walk out of this hospital in exactly six months."

First he practiced drinking on his own. He choked at first, but he kept working at it until he could do it. Then he practiced eating until he could manage by himself. And when the six months were up, the hospital personnel pushed him in a wheelchair—a legal necessity— and at the hospital entrance, he stood up and walked out.

When you refuse to accept the impossible, all things are possible. Maybe these possibilities are what God calls miracles.

Potential of our minds

The human imagination is another miracle. Consider this: We only use ten percent of our brain. And yet, even with this paltry ten percent, look how far we've come. The human being is the only creature on earth who can use creative imagination—brain power—to achieve success. Our imagination is undoubtedly our most valuable asset. Napoleon has been quoted as saying, "Imagination rules the world." And Einstein said, "Imagination *is* the world."

Ninety percent of our brain sits idle! Imagine the possibilities if we could tap into all this potential. Successful people stimulate their minds and their imaginations to reach new goals. They use their brains to mold their internal life, thus creating a more satisfying external life.

It's unfortunate so many parents scold their children for daydreaming. We should encourage our children to use their precious imaginations! The more life they create in their minds, the more mindfully they create their own lives—now and in the future. With enough imagining, maybe we can wake up another percent of our brain power, and then another, and another…

Shake it up!

Mind-numbing routine and stagnation are imagination's greatest enemies. Of course, we need certain routines to make sense of our day-to-day lives (for example, it wouldn't make much sense to shower after I got dressed), but we can make our routines lively and exhilarating. Let's add some flair to our daily activities, infuse them with joy, shake up our routine and chip away at our limits.

When I wake up in the morning, I could glower at my reflection in the mirror as I shave. That's what I used to do, and it wasn't much fun. Now when I wake up, I put on some really rousing songs like *"Celebration"* or *"YMCA."* Then I repeat "yes" a thousand times before I start my day: "yes" in the shower, "yes" as I'm shaving, "yes" as I'm picking out a tie. (It can get a little difficult to keep saying "yes" while I'm eating breakfast, so when my mouth is full, I just say it mentally.) All these "yeses" generate a thousand positive strokes.

I also tell myself—usually in the shower—"I feel happy, I feel healthy, I feel terrific!"

Another thing I do (before the shower) is dance and run naked through my house. I know that sounds a little unusual, but that's the point. I don't want to be trapped in the usual routine. I want to be enlivened. And dancing naked to greet the day, shouting "yes" to welcome new opportunities, telling myself how happy I am—that does the trick for me. By the time I leave the house, my blood is racing.

17

You may choose something different: a certain posture, a particular fragrance, "power clothing," or a specific touch. However, if you decide to try the "naked dance," you might want to close the drapes so the neighbors don't complain.

Anchor points

We face a lot of situations that can make us feel stuck: compulsory meetings, mandatory family obligations, or that seemingly endless line at the Division of Motor Vehicles. How do you "blast" yourself out of these brain-deadening experiences? How do you enliven yourself when you can't dance around naked without being put into a straight jacket? (Straight jackets, I have been told, are extremely limiting.) I'd like to share a couple of ideas.

I've attended a number of seminars where they taught us how to use touch and other anchor points. If you have a very powerful and positive experience, and you anchor it, it will stay with you for life if you reinforce it often enough.

What exactly is anchoring? In *Unlimited Power*, author Tony Robbins describes it as "a sensory stimulus linked to a specific set of states." An anchor may be a word, phrase, touch, or object.

Robbins explains that there are two steps in anchoring a certain feeling. First, you must put yourself into the state you wish to anchor. At the peak of this feeling, you need to provide a unique stimulus. Whenever you use this stimulus in the future, you will revive that feeling.

For example, when you're feeling confident, you're more likely to stand taller, with shoulders back and head held high. Confidence is the state, and posture is the stimulus. When you need to feel that way again, you can do so by adopting a straight, self-assured posture. The rest will follow.

Use anchors carefully

Of course, this also works for negative experiences, so we need to be careful what we anchor. For example, if your father has just died, friends and relatives may come to you and put their arms around you and tell you how sorry they are. That simple gesture has anchored the experience for you. Perhaps a year later, someone comes up to you and puts an arm around you in that same way, and suddenly you feel very sorrowful and you're not sure why. It's because that gesture, that anchor point, brought back the way you felt just after losing one of the most important people in your life.

How anchoring works for me

Fortunately, we can choose to anchor joyous and exhilarating experiences in our lives. For example, one way I've pushed my own limits is by trying things I never did before, such as skydiving. When I jumped out of that airplane at 5,000 feet up, it was an unbelievable experience. You can't believe what that feels like unless you've already done it. I kept shouting "yes, yes yes!" as I floated toward the earth, swinging in the wind. I "anchored" the experience. Now, when I tell myself "yes," it triggers that sense of freedom and amazement; a part of me is still soaring through the air.

I also tried firewalking. I walked across 45 feet of hot coals and I was fired up in more ways than one. I anchored that feeling of excitement, the sense that there wasn't anything I couldn't do. Now, when I'm faced with a challenge, I tap into the firewalk and I'm immediately flooded with the incredible, triumphant feeling that comes with conquering pain and fear.

I have anchor points for joy, for laughter, for freedom, for hope. These all give me the strength I need to keep pushing the limits. I know for a fact that the more I can shatter my limits, the more possibilities I'll discover. The same is true for you, too.

5

Desire, search, and believe

To transform your dream into a tangible, concrete reality, you must really want it to happen. That may sound simple, but if you're going to commit yourself to a goal, you can't do it half-heartedly—you've got to throw yourself into it, be willing to sweat blood to get it.

When you want a goal with everything you've got, then it's already yours. It may not be yours physically or visibly, but you have claimed it. The rest is inevitable.

Ask, seek, and find

Of course, dreams aren't going to land in your lap without some action on your part. If you spend your days watching soap operas, eating chocolates, and picking lint off your sweater, you may not be on the right track for great achievement.

The Bible says, "Ask and you shall receive. Knock and the door will be opened to you. Seek and you shall find." One of my employees pointed out that "A" stands for ask, "S" stands for seek, and "K" stands for knock. If you're disappointed because you're not getting what you want out of life, maybe you need to ask for it, to go out and look for it.

I've heard that luck is the point at which preparation and opportunity intersect. If you want to take advantage of opportunities, you have to be ready for them, you have to be open to them. In other words, turn off the TV, throw away the chocolates, get a new sweater, and embrace the possibilities.

Power of belief

When our beliefs are confident and optimistic, they work in our favor. When our beliefs are dark and limiting, they work against us.

Of course, we didn't necessarily choose the beliefs we started out with. Our belief system has been influenced by parents, teachers, friends, and the media. Our mothers and fathers were probably not even aware of the multitude of beliefs they passed on, just as we may not realize all the beliefs we hand down to our own children. Some beliefs are good and necessary—like believing you should treat others as you would like to be treated—but some of them are pointless and wrong.

For example, it's likely that most of our parents believed grains and carbohydrates had to be the centerpiece of a well-balanced meal. They probably learned it from their parents, who learned it from their parents, and so on. Today, however, we're learning that there are alternative—and perhaps healthier—sources of protein, iron, trace minerals, and B vitamins, and that we can eat a wholesome diet with little or no grains and no carbohydrates except those that come from fruits and vegetables. Our diets require essential amino acids and essential fatty acids but there are no essential carbohydrates.

We also inherit many beliefs about things that are "bad." For example, your father may have had a deathly fear of snakes and you grew up believing that all snakes were dangerous and slimy. Despite any evidence that snakes are mostly harmless and not slimy at all, you may still react to them with revulsion. However, if you grew up with no preconceived fear of snakes, you might even own one as a pet.

Beliefs can change reality

Here are a few more true stories that illustrate the power of belief:

At a baseball game, the administrators had reason to suspect the concession stand of selling contaminated food. Over the public address system, they warned people not to eat that food, as they feared it could cause food poisoning. Most of the people who'd already eaten the food suddenly felt ill. Later, it was discovered that the food was all right, after all. Miraculously, the "sick" people were abruptly well again.

Researchers gave one group of individuals a powerful sedative, and told them it was a strong stimulant and that they would experience more energy than they ever thought possible. The result? They were brimming with vitality, despite this strong drug in their systems.

Conversely, another group was given a potent stimulant, and told it was a strong sedative. Not surprisingly, they went to sleep.

Placebos are 38 to 58 percent effective. When people believe it's going to cure them, it often does. Belief creates results.

21

Restructuring beliefs

To get rid of destructive old beliefs, we need to create constructive new beliefs. And this takes lots of work and practice. You must recite these new beliefs to yourself over and over, until they have finally settled in and made themselves at home, until they truly saturate every corner of your psyche.

It might take years to completely revise your belief system. Be persistent and never, never, never give up. Keep telling yourself, "I believe I will reach an appropriate weight," "I believe I will get the promotion I deserve," or "I believe I am capable, intelligent, and lovable."

Winners believe they will attain the life they want. And when you believe that, you become a winner, too.

Christ's miracles

Jesus Christ was a winner who knew the power of belief. He understood that faith was believing something without any proof. All of Christ's miracles were based on belief. A Centurion once came to Christ and said, "My slave is sick. Can you heal him?" Jesus answered, "I will come." The Centurion said, "No, you don't have to. I know that if you just say so, he will be healed." Christ said, "Never have I seen so much faith." Of course, the slave was healed even though Jesus was nowhere near him.

You may not have a high degree of faith at first. So you work on it with affirmations, visualizations, and the way you use the language. You build up faith. And you'll find that the more faith you have, the more miracles come your way.

My own beliefs

I believe a lot of things, and I am entirely confident they will happen. For example, before our new facility, EuroPharma, in Green Bay, Wisconsin, was built, I knew exactly what it would look like. This was a brand new facility which I envisioned would create a whole new line of natural, innovative and proprietary formulations. Envisioning is one of the keys in accomplishing your dreams. If you can see it and believe it you will receive it. In my mental movie before the ground was even broke, I saw our employees busy throughout the building. I saw the building in my mind exactly the way I wanted it constructed. And now, everything is exactly as I pictured it. Yes, you're right, an architect would have done exactly the same thing, but in order to accomplish our dreams, we must become the architect of our dreams and future.

Our team over the past 30 years had built several natural food retail outlets and a highly successful nutritional manufacturing company. Today, we are building a new research and development facility which will distribute highly effective and clinically studied nutritional products all over the world. We are now in a brand new facility but I believe, in fact I know we will have a 50,000-square-foot addition within the next three years. I can see it already: I know where the manufacturing equipment will be placed throughout the building, and I know how the inventory will be organized and ready for shipping, I know where all the work stations will be placed. Right now, I'm picturing two semi trucks from UPS backed up to the door, being loaded every day, and shipping out cartons of EuroPharma products all over the world. Why do I spend so much time and effort envisioning this process? Because I can't predict the future but I can create it. Whatever we focus on continuously and consistently will become our reality. Most people are where they are in life because of their past thoughts, beliefs and lack of vision. Without a vision we would be like a ship leaving port without a captain riding the high waves without a destination that would more than likely cause the ship to flounder and end up as a disaster. Sounds like the lives of some people who never plan and envision their future.

When I tell people about things that haven't happened yet, I'm not exaggerating—I'm just telling the truth in advance. That's what faith is. You can't see it but you just know it's going to happen the way you planned it. That's the faith that's necessary to accomplish your goals.

God's timing

To reach your dreams, you need to believe in yourself, your supporters, your family, your associates, and God. When you know God is going to help you work things out, you have nothing to worry about. Your goal may not happen exactly when you want it, or exactly how you want it, so you just have to trust in God's timing and wisdom.

We humans are an impatient lot, and I know that at times I'm one of the worst. However, we have to accept that God's pace may be different from ours. All you have to do is know what you want, believe that it's yours, and be open to opportunity. It will come. You won't have to worry about the how's and where's and why's. You'll start to see things happening; it's like a miracle. People will come out of the woodwork to help you. Sometimes I'll be thinking about one of my goals, and all-of-a-sudden somebody will call me up and say, "Hey, I've got a brand-new product and it's fantastic! Do you want to market it for me?" And in fact, that's precisely what I was looking for.

There is someone out there listening to us. When you start thinking about your goal, you are sending a message out into the universe. And the universe always answers.

6

Never quit! Never fear!

Most of us give up much too easily. We fail once or twice and we decide it's because we just can't do it. Who knows what we might accomplish if we never stopped trying?

For example, the man we know as Colonel Sanders had persistence to spare. Before his fame and fortune, he was facing a $99 monthly Social Security income when he retired. He realized he needed to make some more money.

Colonel Sanders wasn't especially brilliant, he never went to college, and he wasn't particularly young or energetic. However, he had two important advantages: a unique chicken recipe and remarkable tenacity.

He said to himself, "Whenever we make this chicken recipe, everybody says it's fantastic, so good it's unbelievable." So Colonel Sanders tried to sell it to a restaurant. The owner said, "Get out of here; we're not going to pay you for that." He got a similar response at the second restaurant. And the third, fourth, fifth, sixth, thirtieth, five-hundredth, and thousandth restaurants. Finally, after approaching over a thousand restaurants, someone agreed to try the recipe.

The rest, of course, is history. Colonel Sanders changed the way people ate. I can't say I admire this kind of deep-fried, fast-food diet, but I do respect the man's amazing persistence and accomplishment.

I had to be persistent, too, during those early years when people poked fun at me for being a "quack" and a "health food nut." Now nutrition and supplements are making headline news; everybody's interested. Recently, a woman I hadn't seen in several years approached me and said, "So you're in the vitamin business. You managed to be in the right place at the right time." I thought to myself, "I've been doing this for 40 years! I was right here the whole time!" But it took almost that long for people to recognize the value of the health food industry and natural approaches to good health.

If you stray off course, get back on

We all get off track from time to time. Our lives are filled with responsibilities and distractions and it's easy to lose focus. When you're folding laundry, watching your children, and answering the phone all at the same time, it's tough to get to that novel you've always wanted to write.

Don't kick yourself for occasionally losing your way. It's easy to do. In fact, did you know that when an airplane flies from California to Hawaii—with a pilot, co-pilot, and navigator—it's usually on course only about 5 percent of the time? The other 95 percent, the crew keeps adjusting and redirecting. Even when they don't stay exactly on track, the crew members never lose sight of their goal. And because their focus is constant—even when their journey isn't—they finally get to where they're supposed to be.

Once you set your goal, your mind constantly directs your self-talk, thoughts, and mental pictures to support it. Use this information— whether positive or negative—to adjust your decisions along the way. Like the airplane crew, you'll eventually reach your destination.

Be open to unexpected possibilities

Keep dreaming. You can still plan to run the Boston Marathon—or whatever your goal is—despite overwhelming distractions. In fact, life's little side trips often open up surprising opportunities.

For example, a dear friend of mine, Dr. Jan McBarron, has a very successful bariatric practice in Georgia, but her dream was to reach as many people as possible all across this country, and not just in Georgia. Together with her husband, Duke, they started off slowly reaching people locally with a very successful radio show called, "Duke and the Doctor". But, there was much more to their dream. Their dream was to reach as many people across the country suffering from illness and disease. Dr. McBarron, a highly skilled alternative physician, had great empathy for many people who had been prescribed medications but were looking for a more natural and safer alternative. Their dream is not even close to being finished but they are well on their way to accomplishing their goals. Their show is a 2 hour radio program that offers nutritional advice and ways to work with conventional doctors to reduce the number of prescription drugs. They have made a huge impact on helping improve the health of America and this all came about because of the many questions that Dr. McBarron was asked by her patients. That sparked an unexpected possibility that maybe there are hundreds of thousands of people just like her patients. Now there is a daily "Duke and the Doctor" radio show reaching almost every city in the United States. Duke and the Doctor had compassion and the good sense to embrace this new opportunity.

Failure? No such thing

I truly believe there is no such thing as failure. There are only results. Everything happens for a reason.

When you face a challenge, see what you can learn from it. Discover what you can use from your mistakes. For example, one of my staff writers creates fiction in her spare time. When something unfortunate occurs, she turns it into a story. She transforms negative experiences into art. That way, nothing goes to waste.

Watch out for so-called "sympathizers"

Like Colonel Sanders, we've all faced setbacks. What happens when you hit a rough spot? Unfortunately, you may unwittingly attract a certain breed of individual who thrives on the failures of others. Why? Because misery loves company. These kind of people don't want to see you succeed. They like the inertia—the comfort—of not doing anything to improve their lives, and they want you right down there with them. They're afraid to see you make something of your life because they don't want to go nowhere alone. When you stumble, they pretend to be sympathetic but they're secretly relieved.

Avoid these people! Instead, seek out friends who encourage you to reach your highest goals and become the best person you can be. Find people who help you move forward when you falter. They'll support you as you reach your full potential. These are your real friends; they'll celebrate your successes because they're not threatened by them. They truly want the best for you.

The deeper the valley, the higher the peak

Of course, a positive attitude can't prevent tragedy. Some tragedy in life is inevitable. Parents die. Marriages break up. Children disappoint us. But I am convinced that when God closes one door, he opens two others. In every adversity, you can find a seed of opportunity.

I also believe that you can't have a peak unless you have a valley. And the peak is going to be as high as the valley is low. No matter how deep a gully I walk through, I know the peak is on the other side. There would have been no Resurrection without the Crucifixion. When we think of Christ's suffering, we also have to remember the incredible miracle that followed. When you face profound tragedy, always remember that your own miracle is just around the corner. That realization will get you through some dark times.

I once heard about an insurance salesman who took nine months to sell his first policy. Any other person might have given up—seen only the valley without anticipating the peak. But this man stuck with it. I'm certain he became disappointed, but he knew better times were ahead. And in fact, three years after he sold his first policy, he retired a millionaire. You may not retire a millionaire, but you can still succeed.

Everything happens for good

It's been my experience over the years that everything that happens is for the best. It may seem bad at the time because we don't understand it. For example, it's natural to perceive a divorce as shattering and heartbreaking. But in the years ahead, you may realize that both you and your partner are living better lives, separately.

Losing a job can momentarily crush your self-esteem. But it also frees you up to find out what you truly want to do, to discover work that you feel a genuine passion for. If you hadn't been laid off, you might never have found your true calling.

God knows the answer

When I talk about God, it isn't because I'm trying to "convert" anyone or take the moral upper hand. It's just that God is the most important aspect of my life. I owe everything to God: my health, my family, my business, my friends. It's impossible to write about my philosophies without including God.

When we trust God, we can endure. This is true for me, and you're very fortunate if it's true for you, too. Without God, we're like a raft in the middle of the ocean, thrown about helplessly with every passing wind, splintered by the first violent storm. God doesn't take away the storms, but He does give us the fortitude to weather the worst.

Life hands us our share of disappointments and tragedies. I have been through them myself: I helped care for my father as he died of a painful and lingering illness. I have endured family crises and lost friends. I have faced setbacks in my business.

Having a positive attitude helps us make the most out of life, but it does not shield us from all of life's disappointments. God does not shield us from life's disappointments, either, but He does help us understand them and grow from them.

I talk to God a lot. When I'm faced with a challenge, I seek His help. "What am I supposed to learn from this?" I ask. "What changes should I make? In one way or another, God always sends an answer.

For example, while God did not spare me from my father's difficult death, He gave me an opportunity to become more compassionate to the suffering of others. God did not protect me from the loss of important relationships, but He taught me to nurture my family ties and friendships with greater love and attention. And God did not prevent my occasional business setback, but He helped me learn from them and build an even stronger business as a result.

God's in the driver's seat

Have you ever seen one of those strap-in car seats with the attached toy steering wheel? The baby or toddler turns the steering wheel this way and that, convinced he or she is actually driving the car. Sometimes I think we're a little like that. We're put in our "baby seat" here on earth, convinced that every aspect of our journey here is under our control. And all along, God is truly the one in the driver's seat.

Am I saying we have no free will? Of course not. I am saying that when we turn our lives over to God, He gives us the opportunity to choose the best direction. For example, God gives us all 24 hours a day, and He allows us to use them as we choose. When we're tuned in to God, He guides us to use this time to help others, to accomplish something constructive, to work on self-improvement. Without God, we may squander our time in self-centered pursuits or sloth.

God's in the driver's seat, but He still lets us do plenty of navigating. If we just listen to Him, we'll reach our destination.

7

God's in charge—thank God!

When we grow up, we get our own car and our own house and our own family and maybe even our own business. And sometimes we make the mistake of believing we're totally in control of our lives. Guess what? We're not. God is. And paradoxically, the more of our lives we turn over to God, the more truly empowered we become.

God is our Father, a loving parent who wants only the best for us. The Bible tells us that God takes care of the sparrows and the lilies, and he will certainly take care of us.

If you're a parent, you know the challenges you face every day. On the one hand, you want to protect your child from unpleasantness and failure. On the other hand, you know your child needs to take risks, to perhaps stumble occasionally along the path to adulthood and independence. You know that if you shelter your child from every responsibility, he or she is likely to end up spoiled, self-centered, and not particularly likable.

God faces the same choices with us. He doesn't just leave us to flounder, but He does allow us to make mistakes we can learn from.

Power of trust

"Mistakes," however, often have a way of working out for the best. I believe things happen for a reason, although it may not always be obvious. Sometimes we don't understand why we have to face certain challenges, but God understands. We need to trust that God, our wise and loving parent, knows what we need to experience to become the kind of people He knows we can be.

I have a certain affirmation that I repeat to myself several times a day, that helps keep me anchored: "All things good happen to those who love the Lord."

God didn't tell us that *some* things happen for good, or 25 good things happen per person, or three good things per year. He said *all* things happen for good. So if I believe in and love the Lord, I have to trust that what He's telling me is true. Sometimes it's not easy, but we can't expect it to be easy: We're not born of the spirit; we're born of the world.

Importance of faith

Faith is a tough concept. Most of us want hard proof; tangible, concrete facts. Western intellectual tradition teaches us to question everything, to accept nothing without solid evidence. And in the world of facts and figures and business dealings and bottom lines, that's a smart rule to live by. But in the spiritual realm, in God's Kingdom, we don't need to question. We just believe.

If you have faith, nothing is impossible to you. Nothing. If you believe you will receive whatever you ask for in prayer, it shall be done for you.

Now, it won't necessarily happen exactly the way you imagined. You might pray for riches and never make much money. Instead, you may enjoy a wealth of love and encouragement from family, friends, co-workers, and neighbors. You might pray that you marry a beautiful person. You could end up falling in love with someone who falls short of the physical ideal, but whose generosity, kindness, and wisdom makes him or her the most beautiful person you've ever met.

We may think we know what we want, but God knows what we need.

Due season

A young man once asked God, "How much money do you have?" God said, "I have all the money in the world, my son." The man asked, "Well, what's a million dollars to You?" God answered, "It's like a penny." The man then asked, "How old are you?" God said, "I've been around since the beginning of time." The man asked, "What is a hundred years to you?" God said, "It's about a second." The man thought about this for a while, and then said, "Give me a million dollars, then." And God answered, "I will, in just a second."

The point of the story, of course, is that God's time is different than our time. He has a time and season for everything. Farmers understand this. They don't plant their seeds and then go home at night and think, "I wonder if those seeds will come up. I bet they won't; I probably planted those seeds for nothing. I bet I'm too fat to plant seeds. I bet I'm too dumb to plant seeds. I don't have a college education, so I can't plant seeds."

It is our nature to be impatient. We plant a seed and then we want to pick up the ground to see what's going on. If we don't see immediate results from our efforts, we feel like a failure. Our only failure is not trusting that our goals will come to fruition when the time is right.

The farmer knows that crops grow and mature in due season. He plants in good faith, just as we need to plant our own seeds in good faith.

Our goals are small seeds with the potential for great bounty. We plant them into the universe, and the universe returns a rich harvest of opportunity. It may not happen in an instant—perhaps not for years—but it will happen. God knows when it's time, and He will tell us.

If you dream it, you can have it

We all have dreams. I dream of improving the health of people around the world with natural products. You may dream of finding the cure for cancer, or buying a home of your own, or losing weight, or getting a Ph.D. Unfortunately, we often scold ourselves for dreaming. It's that self-destructive, negative self-talk: "Who am I to run an international business?" "I'll never be able to afford my own home." "I've never been able to lose weight; why should this time be any different?" "I'm not smart enough to get a Ph.D."

If you dream it, you can do it. God wouldn't give you a dream if you couldn't achieve it. The possibility wouldn't even occur to you. God only gives you attainable dreams. So don't tell yourself you can't do something when God knows you can.

The more you give, the more you get

Jesus Christ gives us an important message: In order to receive, we must give. If you say, "I wish I had a friend," try *being* a friend—you'll be amazed by the friendship that comes your way. If you say, "I wish I had more love in my life," try giving away love—it will come back to you many times over.

Whatever we give comes back multiplied, whether it's love, our talents, or our money. By giving, we create a vacuum in the universe, and that vacuum has to be filled. And it will be filled by *more* than what we gave away. So, if you need money, try giving it away (preferably to people who have a legitimate need for it). If you need help, start helping others. If you start giving, people will give back to you, over and over.

Tithing

To tithe is to give 10 percent of your money to a worthy, charitable organization. Choose something you believe in: your church, Salvation Army, Literacy Council, hospice—whatever is important to you.

Tithing represents one of the greatest financial laws in the universe: Whatever you give, you get more back. And don't wait until the end of the month to see what you've got left. Take 10 percent at the beginning of the month. You might say, "Good Lord, I won't have enough at the end of the month!" I know that; that's why you need to give some away. Because when you give, your whole life is going to change. Believe me, it works.

God said, "Trust Me, or test Me, and see if I'm not true to My word, that if you give and you tithe, I will open the heavens and pour out great blessings." God gives us seeds to sow, not to store up.

All things are possible

I don't consider myself a professional writer, but I created this book because I very much want to share my message. It's not actually from me; it's from many other writers, thinkers, and the Holy Bible. I'm just trying to simplify it and make it more accessible.

I honestly believe that when we live by a certain philosophy, all the details fall into place. When we keep sight of the "big picture," the small stuff takes care of itself.

Sure, life can present us with plenty of challenges. Having a strong, positive philosophy doesn't make hardships go away. But it does transform them into opportunities for growth, compassion, and wisdom.

The thought I want to leave you with is this: Your mind and spirit are your most powerful assets. When you nourish these, you empower yourself. You discover all the incredible miracles that are truly within your grasp.

Everything is possible when you believe.